Toning Your Life
Use Your Voice to Enhance Your Health

Justine Bauer
2015

Toning Your Life: Use Your Voice to Enhance Your Health

To contact the author, visit
http://justine-bauer.healthcoach.integrativenutrition.com/

ISBN-13: 978-1511576406

ISBN-10: 1511576405
Printed in the United States of America

Toning Your Life:
Use Your Voice to Enhance Your Health

Table of Contents

Dedication

At times our own
light goes out and is
rekindled by a spark
from another.

Albert Schweitzer

I have been fortunate in my life to have encountered and
been given support by many wonderful people.
My sincerest thanks to all.

Acknowledgements

As a new author of a first book I'm finding that I want to thank everyone and I'm afraid I'm going to forget many. I'd like to start by offering thanks to my brother, Peter Collins and his wife Catherine P. Collins, my parents, Olga and Peter Collins, and my grandparents Juliana and Thomas Kameika. Along with them, I'd like to include in my thanks all of my aunts and uncles, cousins, relatives and friends that were so important to me when I was growing up. Every person and institution I think of leads to more people and places that have helped me throughout my life and therefore have contributed to this project in some way. Even those who seemed less than helpful at the time, have made positive contributions toward my progress, albeit without their knowledge and intentions. The list is infinite, so here's the beginning...

Mike Bauer, my husband who does everything and is my greatest support

Rob and Alice Adams, my son and his wife who bring joy to my life

Angela Bauer, the first to read my book twice and tell me how much she loved it

Terri Bauer, who took time during her busy college schedule to make notes in my manuscript

Marc Wohl, a new friend who offered to help with editing

Kathryn Grieco, who volunteered Marc

Nancy Osborn, who offers inspiration and support

Lois Rosenberg Brown, my book writing buddy who kept me on track

Leslie Ayd, someone to talk with about anything

Marian Sanborn, who helps me to expand my dreams

Ursula Brown, who travelled with me to California

Optimum Health Institute, a lovely place in California

Marie Cantu DC, who tries to keep me well adjusted

Nicole Cutler LAC, who taught me to breathe

PS 71, Hunter College HS, Hunter College, my formal education

Access SFL, a workplace that has been a source of friends

Natural Gourmet Institute, cooking that's still ahead of its time

Song of the Valley Chorus, a welcoming group of barber-shoppers who let me sing with them

Lindsey Smith, inspiration for authors

Joshua Rosenthal and Institute of Integrative Nutrition, man with a vision and a plan

Peter Mark Roget, whose thesaurus was a wonderful idea

And if you're reading this, put your name here: _____

Introduction

If you're reading this book, or considering it, it's possible that you're someone who knows me or you're someone who is looking for "something." Perhaps you're trying to find better health or balance in your life. Maybe you're bored with your usual routine and are interested in trying something a little different. It just may be that you didn't know you were looking for or missing anything, and this book crossed your path creating a spark of interest and a space and opportunity to experience something new. Something very similar happened to me.

A few years ago I travelled with a friend to California to spend a week at the Optimum Health Institute, eating raw foods and drinking wheatgrass and juices. There were also opportunities for massage and colonics as well as daily exercise classes. To encourage and assist people in making positive lifestyle changes and exploring new interests to continue at home, demonstrations and lectures were also available. Some of the topics included "the benefits of a raw diet," "dehydrating foods," "additives to avoid," and "toning."

I had never heard of "toning" and had no expectations. A facilitator and a recording guided our group through a series of vocalizations combined with visualizations. As the session progressed, I became aware of both physical sensations and a spiritual experience. By the end of our session I felt that toning was a very powerful "group experience" and I was interested in having it again.

I returned home, and guided by my misconceptions I started looking for a "toning group." Most of the people I contacted had not heard of toning, there were no groups to join, and I didn't find anyone interested in forming a group. Eventually, I moved on to other things.

Recently, I encountered toning again. Ironically, in the reading I've done so far, there's no mention of groups being important or even necessary to the process. I've been excited to learn that the benefits of toning can be experienced by an individual and is not reliant on the energy of a group. I can practice toning by myself whenever I want. And so can you! Enjoy!

Chapter 1
Energy Centers and Toning

Singing daily for at least ten minutes
reduces stress,
clears sinuses,
improves posture
and can even
help you live longer

David Avocado Wolfe

Toning is not exactly singing but it can provide the same benefits mentioned above and more. It can contribute to physical, mental and spiritual wellbeing. The regular practice of toning can be used as a preventive measure or in support of other healing disciplines. Toning can be done almost anywhere, with or without special equipment, alone or in a group. Simply put, toning involves using your voice to create balance in your life. And just like singing, toning can be fun!

The basis of toning is the belief that all things are composed of energy and everything has a specific optimal vibration or frequency. This idea is a little abstract for some of us. Although we can hear sounds, we don't ordinarily think about the vibrations and frequencies used to create them. However, they can be measured scientifically and the explanation of our ability to hear involves vibrations within our ears. Sometimes we can feel or see the results of sound vibrations. Remember when the sound of thunder shook the house, when the music at the concert shook the seats, or when the operatic soprano shattered the crystal champagne flute with her voice during the classic movie scene?

The same is true for light and other forms of energy. Many of us don't think about colors and frequencies as being related. If we're fortunate, we appreciate their beauty. Most of us can feel the heat from a radiator or stove and have seen a hot air balloon floating through the sky, lifted by heat and propelled by currents of air. Some people can see or feel energy or auras of other people or objects and Kirilian photography can be used as a type of visual energy measure.

The belief that there are energy centers related to the physical, mental, and spiritual aspects of a person dates back to ancient times. Disciplines such as Ayurveda, Acupuncture, Chiropractic, Yoga, and Tai Chi are only a few of the practices that can involve a holistic relationship of mind, body, and spirit and the flow of energy.

It is thought that there are seven major energy centers in the body commonly referred to as "chakras'. These centers are sometimes thought of as "wheels of energy". The first center is located at the base of the spine. The others are positioned at intervals above, with the seventh being located at the top of the head. There are also thought to be other minor energy centers including some that are located outside the body.

Many of our traditional health, religious and cultural systems include guidelines for daily living as well as rituals and protocols for special occasions or circumstances. These instructions often involve foods and drinks to eat or avoid, either on a regular basis or during specific times. There are specific herbs and plants recommended to be ingested or burned for healing and cleansing of the body and the physical world or connecting to the spiritual. Incense used in churches and smudging are two examples. And it seems as though almost every culture includes music, not only for entertainment but also related to healing and spirituality. Examples include religious chanting and hymns as well as Native American shamanic rituals.

Toning can also be enhanced by including certain foods and drinks. For some of us it's easy to believe that the colorful foods we were told to eat as children are healthy because of phytonutrients and less easy to believe in their energetic properties. But phytonutrients are newly discovered compared to our ancestral beliefs that including a variety of foods in one's diet is important for health. Also beneficial are herbs, aromas, and essential oils.

Focusing on the colors associated with each chakra can also help to align the energies. Stones, gems and crystals either in the form of jewelry or chakra kits are available and can provide vibrational support as well. Not all sources, cultures or healing systems are in agreement as to which items are the best choices for balance and healing. It is important to remember that each of us has our own "bio-individuality" and must rely on our own body, mind and spirit to guide us.

Chapter 2
Toning Basics

Toning can be done while sitting or standing. If sitting, choose a comfortable position in a chair or on the ground. Either sitting or standing, it's important to keep the spine aligned to allow the energy to flow freely, the airways to remain open and the lungs to expand and contract efficiently.

The notes to use when toning suggested later in this book are the music notes "C" through "B". They are available at http://justine-bauer.healthcoach.integrativenutrition.com/ A pitch pipe, musical instrument or cellphone app might also be convenient. Some people use chakra bowls or tuning forks. Others recommend Solfeggio frequencies or hertz frequencies to achieve maximum compatibility for balance and healing. Still others believe that specific notes and frequencies are unimportant. Try choosing a comfortable lower note to start and raise the notes as you move upward through the energy centers. Perhaps, listening to your own body and setting intentions of health and balance are most important. Having a determined mindset that includes definite goals and expectations can only help to attract positive energies.

Also a matter of personal choice, perhaps influenced by time constraints, is the length of time allotted for toning each energy center and how often toning is practiced. Try starting with three breaths for each note. Experiment with increasing the number of breaths or using a timer. Toning practice can be easily adjusted to individual needs and practiced daily, a few times a week, or as needed. Just as with exercise and meditation routines, toning can be abbreviated when time is short and expanded when time permits. As with most healing or preventive disciplines, consistency may provide greater benefits. However, toning can also be used successfully to increase a sense of balance with the change of seasons or when special circumstances occur. Again, listen to your body.

If you like to have a way to measure outcomes, and especially if you are planning to use toning as part of a solution for a specific challenge, you might consider keeping a journal. It does not need to be complicated, but it can help to track changes and sometimes highlight benefits and progress that might otherwise have been overlooked.

grounding

"uh"

Chapter 3
"Grounding" Energy Center

Overview

The energy center that is considered to be the first or foundation is located near the base of the spine. It is known as the "root" chakra. This center is associated with instinct, safety, fear and survival. It is also thought to be connected to family and security. If you believe in "spiritual genetics" this center would be where your ancestral history is stored and may be connected to intergenerational family traits. For the physical body this center can be associated with the spinal column, kidneys, legs, feet, rectum, adrenals and immune system. It is not surprising that this is the "grounding" center. And although overall balance of energies is important, as the base, this may be a starting point or a place that needs special attention.

Toning

The tone for the "root" center is the music note "C" combined with the vowel sound "uh" as in cup.

Focusing on the base of the spine while viewing or imagining the color "red" can enhance the toning experience for this energy center. Crystals, gemstones and aromas that could be included in the toning of this center might include hematite, garnet or smoky quartz and cedar or patchouli. Go outside every day and feel the ground under your feet whenever possible as this energy center is connected to the earth. Think, "I am strong, I am secure, I am healthy, I am prosperous!"

Recipe

Another wonderful and delicious balancing tool is food. Not surprisingly, food choices that may fortify this energy center include root vegetables such as beets, carrots and sweet potato and red-colored foods like pomegranate, apple, and radish.

Mushrooms and protein, especially animal protein may also be beneficial. Below is a recipe that nourishes this grounding energy center and also seems like "comfort food."

Roasted Root Vegetables

The great thing about this recipe is that it's very flexible. I usually have many of these vegetables on hand and so the proportions are different depending on my mood and what's available. And I always use my largest roasting pan and enjoy the leftovers. Please add in or leave out ingredients to your taste.

Choose a pan that will allow the vegetables to be tossed and not crowded. The vegetables will be stirred both before cooking and during cooking when the pan will be hot.

Ingredients:

- Root vegetables, washed and peeled and cut into 1 inch pieces (use sweet potatoes, potatoes, carrots, parsnips, turnips, rutabagas, beets) - *if you're purchasing vegetables, start with about 2 pounds; otherwise, add a variety to the pan being careful not to overcrowd; if using organic and you enjoy the skin, it can be left on but remember that some vegetable skin, such as carrot can be bitter*
- 1 medium-large onion cut into wedges sized to match the vegetables
- Olive oil - *start with 1 tablespoon and add in 1 tablespoon at a time until vegetables are lightly coated*
- Salt to taste - *use less and adjust as you eat*
- 1 head garlic, peeled and separated - *or less if it's a large head*
- Jewels of a pomegranate or fresh chopped herbs of choice and/or balsamic vinegar for garnish – *start with a light touch and increase slowly to taste*

Directions:

- Heat oven to 400 degrees - *in warm weather, this recipe can be made on the grill using a vegetable rack; I especially love grilled beets*
- Place the root vegetables and onion in a roasting pan
- Toss with olive oil and salt - *sometimes it's easier to toss in a large food storage bag or put oil in a spray bottle to apply*
- Roast for about 1 hour - stirring and checking about every 15 minutes to prevent burning
- After 30 minutes stir in garlic
- Cook until vegetables are tender and lightly browned or caramelized
- Garnish and serve
- Enjoy!

emotional
"ooh"

Chapter 4
"Emotional" Energy Center

Overview

The second energy center, moving up from the base of the spine, is located in your lower abdomen about one to three inches below the naval. It is known as the "sacral" chakra. This center is associated with emotion, creativity, wisdom, personal expression and sexuality. When thinking of this energetic area the expressions "gut feelings" and 'listen to your gut" come to mind. For the physical body, it is not surprising, based on location, that the body parts connected to this energy center are hips, lower back, sexual organs, bladder, kidneys, stomach, and large intestine. And this center is also linked to liquid - water as well as bodily fluids.

Toning

The musical note for the "emotional" center is "D" and the toning sound would be "ooh" as in "you."

An area below the naval that connects the abdomen and spine would be the physical focal point for this center. The color "orange" is associated with this center and could be imagined or viewed while producing the toning note. Crystals and gemstones to hold or place on the abdomen might consist of amber, coral, orange calcite, or carnelian Aromas that could be included in the toning of this center might include orange/citrus scents, bergamot, cardamom and clary sage. A moonlight walk on the beach might provide the perfect venue to support the sacral chakra, although any exposure to water could be of benefit. Think, "I am joyful, I am creative, I am passionate, I am at peace!"

Recipe

Supporting foods for this energy center include orange colored fruits and vegetables such as tangerines, oranges, carrots, sweet potato, pumpkin, papaya, mango and melon as well as tropical pineapples and coconuts. Fish, especially wild caught salmon, and healthy fats and oils are associated with this center and beneficial flavors include vanilla, cinnamon, carob, nuts and honey.

The following balancing tool for the sacral center provides many opportunities for creativity and adjusting the ingredients to your own pleasure. It looks complicated in writing but the ingredients and techniques are common and not difficult.

Grilled Salmon and Salad with Orange Dressing

This is one of my favorite recipes for salmon. Not only does the mustard add flavor, the coating also keeps the fish moist and provides a little cushion of time in case the cook is distracted by children or the phone or realizes that the platter for the salmon is not nearby. The salmon can be served with a large salad alone or additional sides can be added. If "a little extra" is prepared the leftovers can be thrown together, perhaps with a different dressing, and served cold for lunch the next day. And the dressing can be varied by preparing it in a high speed blender and using chunks of the peeled orange rather than just the juice and adding a splash of champagne vinegar or balsamic vinegar.

Ingredients:

Salmon
- Alaskan or sockeye Salmon - *fresh caught steaks or fillets are best if available but previously frozen can also be used; portion size is usually 4-6 ounces or about the size of the palm of your hand*
- Prepared mustard - *find a Dijon style mustard with as high a seed content as possible*

Salad

- Mixed greens - *choose your favorites or try a new mix, perhaps with kale*
- Carrots, peeled and grated or diced
- Orange pepper, diced
- Cucumber slices – *use organic, local or home grown if using the peel*
- Raw or roasted sesame or pumpkin seeds for garnish

Orange Dressing

- 1 orange - *organic would be best since the rind will be used*
- 2-3 tablespoons lime or lemon juice - *lemon tends to have a stronger flavor*
- Extra virgin olive oil
- Ground coriander - *start with ¼ teaspoon and increase to taste*
- Salt and pepper to taste - *start with a pinch or none*

Directions:

- Rinse and pat dry the salmon
- If using steaks or skinless fillets, coat both sides with mustard remembering not to dip your utensil in the jar if it's touched the fish
- If using fillets with skin, coat only the non-skin side at this time, reserving some mustard to apply later; *again remember to use only a clean utensil in the mustard jar*
- Cover and refrigerate until ready to grill

- Rinse the greens and shake off extra moisture or use a salad spinner and place in a large bowl
- Rinse and prepare the carrot, pepper and cucumber slices and add to the greens
- Garnish with the seeds
- Cover and refrigerate if you like your salad chilled

- Rinse the orange and lime or lemon
- Grate the orange and collect the zest
- Use a reamer to extract the juice from the orange and the lime or lemon juice
- Place the juice in a small jar or small, deep bowl
- Add olive oil; *the usual proportions are for a salad dressing is 1 part acid to 3 parts oil, so start by adding oil equal to the amount of juice and increase to taste*
- Add coriander, salt and pepper
- Cover jar and shake or stir
- Adjust seasonings to taste
- Refrigerate until ready to serve

- Heat and oil the grill – *remember if using an indoor grill and especially one that closes, the cooking surface is actually touching the fish and the cooking time will be less than on an outdoor grill*
- Grilling time for fish is about 10 minutes per inch; check early to avoid overcooking
- **For steaks**, place on grill cooking about ½ the time on each side, turning only once if possible
- **For fillets**, place on grill skin side down for a short time to sear skin
- Turn fillet over and remove skin with a fork
- Coat the now skinless side with mustard; it may be easiest to "rake" it across the surface with a fork
- When the salmon is ready to eat, remove from grill and serve immediately with salad dressed to taste; shake or stir dressing again before use
- Enjoy!

Sweet Potato Quinoa Patties – Vegan Alternative to Grilled Salmon

This recipe can be quickly put together using previously prepared sweet potatoes and quinoa, especially since it is easier to work with the ingredients once they have cooled. The recipe makes about 10 to 12 cakes that can be individually wrapped and frozen for enjoyment at a later time.

Use a greased or parchment lined baking sheet to prepare patties in the oven. The patties can also be cooked on an outdoor grill using a rack or on an indoor grill.

Ingredients:

- 3 medium baked sweet potatoes – *about 3 cups of sweet potato or pumpkin*
- 2 cups cooked quinoa – *or grain of choice*
- 1 flax egg – *mix together 1 tablespoon ground flax seeds or chia seeds with 3 tablespoons of water; allow to set in the refrigerator for at least 15 minutes*
- 2-3 scallions, chopped
- 2-3 cloves garlic, crushed
- ¼ - ½ teaspoon sea salt
- ½ teaspoon paprika
- 1 tsp. cumin
- ¼ teaspoon cinnamon
- 1-2 tablespoons olive oil – *to be used for greasing the baking sheet, outdoor rack or indoor grill; putting a small amount on the hands before forming the patties to prevent sticking; and brushing the patties before cooking*

Directions:

- Preheat oven to 350 degrees
- Place sweet potatoes in a large bowl and mash with a fork. A ricer or potato masher can also be used.

- Stir in quinoa, flax egg, scallions, garlic, salt, and spices until well combined
- Use a ¼ cup measure to scoop mixture, then flatten into patties and place on the prepared baking sheet
- Brush patties with olive oil
- Bake for 15-20 minutes until heated through and golden
- Enjoy!

vitality

"oh"

Chapter 5
"Vitality" Energy Center

Overview

"Solar plexus" is the third energy center travelling upward from the base of the spine. It is associated with the liver, stomach and the gallbladder, as well as the skin and nervous system. This center is connected to personal power, self-confidence, discipline, humor and joy. Balancing the vibrations here can boost self-esteem and self-love contributing to a more positive sense of self-worth. Picture a joyous yellow energy emanating from within.

Toning

The tone for the "solar plexus" center is the music note "E". The vowel sound "oh" as in "go" is used with this note.

While focusing on the area below the breastbone, viewing a picture or imagining the color "yellow" may assist in the toning process. The scents that support this center include rosemary, ginger, juniper, rose and lavender. Amber, citrine, tiger's eye, sunstone and yellow jasper are gemstones that may provide vibrations aligned to this energy center. The sun and fire are associated with this vitality center so outdoor activities on beautiful days and sitting by the fireplace in the evenings seems perfect. "I love and accept myself," "I am strong and courageous," "I choose the best for myself" and "I am authentic" might be affirmations to consider to bolster this center.

Recipe

Yellow foods share the color vibration for this energy center. If the "root" center is considered to be the protein center and the "sacral" center is associated with healthy oils and fats, the "solar plexus" is related to carbohydrates. Consuming healthy carbohydrates is important to maintaining balance. Choose yellow lentils, sweet yellow corn, yellow peppers, legumes, butternut squash and whole grains. Flaxseed and sunflower seeds, chamomile, turmeric, cumin, ginger and fennel also aid this chakra. Tropical fruits such as lemons, bananas, papayas and pineapple are also great to have around.

Yellow Lentils with Coconut Milk

This recipe can be used as a main dish with some steamed vegetables and/or salad or as a side served with a protein of your choice. For the solar plexus energy center grilled lemon chicken might be appropriate. Or use vegetables as the main dish with a side of lentils. Pungent vegetables such as kale and Brussels sprouts complement the slightly sweet taste of the lentils. The recipe freezes well and when reheating, leftover meats and vegetables can be added to quickly create a new dish. Although it might not support the solar plexus center as well, other varieties of lentils can also be used. The cooking times and results will be different, but delightful.

Choose a 6 quart saucepan if one is available. The recipe should also fit in a 4 quart pan but it seems a little scary. A better option might be to sauté the spice mixture in a frying pan and then cook the lentils in a crockpot.

Ingredients:

- 3 cups yellow lentils - *sort and rinse*
- 7 cups water
- 1 large yellow onion, coarsely chopped
- Diced tomatoes - *1/ 14 ounce can, fire roasted are quite nice but any would be fine; or about 1 ¾ cup fresh or grilled diced tomatoes, yellow, red or mixed*
- ½ teaspoon cayenne pepper
- 1 teaspoon ground cumin
- 1 teaspoon ground coriander
- ½ teaspoon ground turmeric

- 1 teaspoon sea salt
- 2 tablespoons coconut oil or ghee
- 2 teaspoons cumin seeds
- 1 teaspoon yellow mustard seeds
- 1 small-medium yellow onion, finely chopped
- Coconut milk, 1/ 14 ounce can
- Sunflower seeds – *raw or toasted*
- Lemon zest

Directions:

- In the saucepan, *or frying pan if using a crockpot*, warm the oil or ghee over medium to high heat.
- When the oil is hot, add the cumin seeds and the mustard seeds.
- Cover the pan and wait briefly until the mustard seeds begin to pop.
- Lower the heat and add the finely chopped onion.
- Cook, stirring constantly to prevent burning, until onion is lightly browned.
- Combine the lentils, coarsely chopped onion, tomatoes, cayenne, ground cumin, coriander, turmeric, and salt in the saucepan *or crockpot*.
- *If using the crockpot, add the spice mixture from the frying pan.*
- Add the 7 cups of water to the saucepan *or crockpot.*
- Bring the saucepan contents to a boil, then lower to a simmer.
- Simmer ½ hour or longer, until lentils are tender.
- *Set the crockpot to "high" for 4 hours.*
- Add coconut milk to the lentil mixture.
- Cook another 10-30 minutes to blend flavors.
- Plate and garnish with a small handful of sunflower seeds and a little lemon zest.
- Enjoy!

loving

"ah"

Chapter 6
"Loving" Energy Center

Overview

The "heart" chakra, which is located in the center of the chest, provides a balance and bridge between the three lower chakras and the three upper. In the physical body, it associated with the heart and lungs as well as to the upper back, blood and circulatory system. This energy center is about unconditional love, connection and acceptance. If this "heart" center is thought of as a center for spirituality, it could be considered a hub for transformation, healing and love and a connection to "all that is."

Toning

The tone for the "heart" center is the music note "F" combined with the vowel sound "ah" as in "ma".

Focusing on the middle of the chest while viewing or imagining the color "green" can enhance the toning experience for this energy center. Crystals and gemstones that could be beneficial in the toning of this center might include rose quartz, emerald, jade and green tourmaline. Rose, tuberose and bergamot may provide support for balancing this center. Being outside and breathing fresh air are supportive of this center, especially when everything is green and lush. "I am compassionate," "I am understanding" and "I am loving" are affirmations to consider.

Recipe

Food choices that may fortify this "green" energy center are abundant. Leafy greens that include kale, spinach, chard, collards, dandelion and mustard greens and lettuce as well as sprouts of all kinds lead the list. Cruciferous vegetables such as broccoli, Brussels sprouts and cauliflower can be supportive to this chakra along with bok choy, cabbage, arugula, green peas and peppers, leeks and green onions, watercress, zucchini, celery, and more. Many of these are easy to grow at home and readily available at local Farmer's Markets and winter CSA's. Green fruits such as green apples, pears, grapes and kiwi and the versatile avocado can be included in your diet. Basil, sage, thyme, cilantro, parsley are just a few of the herbs that can be used to create exciting and delicious meals. And green tea can also be included here.

The ingredients that support the "vitality" energy center are versatile and can be eaten raw or cooked and used to create juices and smoothies. There is such a huge variety that there is always something readily available throughout the year.

Braised Kale

This recipe is quick and easy. It can be made to accompany a more complicated recipe, as part of a quick weeknight dinner or as an addition to leftovers to create a tasty change from the night before. Just add a little more liquid and cook a little longer and it's also a delicious way to prepare broccoli rabe.

Choose a large skillet or wok with a lid. The pan will be very full at first but will cook down quickly allowing room for the entire bunch of kale to be added.

Ingredients:

- 1 large bunch kale – *remove thick stems by stripping them from the leaves or folding the leaves in half cutting them away; tear the leaves into small pieces or chop using a knife; discard the stems or save for juicing or composting; rinse leaves well in a colander remembering that kale can be sandy; drain allowing some of the moisture to remain*
- 3 or more cloves garlic, crushed – *depending on the size of the cloves, the type of garlic you're using and your personal taste, more can be added*
- 2 tablespoons extra virgin olive oil

- ¼-½ teaspoon sea salt – *kelp flakes or soy sauce could be substituted*
- Freshly ground pepper – *grind directly into the pan while cooking*
- ¼-½ cup liquid – *water, chicken broth or miso; if using broth or miso, reduce salt*
- Splash of lemon juice or balsamic vinegar
- Sprinkle of grated cheese or hemp hearts to garnish

Directions:

- Warm the oil over medium heat
- Place the garlic and kale in the pan stirring quickly to mix and prevent sticking and burning
- Add salt and pepper; continue stirring
- Add liquid as needed, cover and lower heat to simmer until kale is tender
- Plate and splash with lemon juice or balsamic vinegar if desired
- Garnish and serve
- Enjoy!

communication
"eye"

Chapter 7
"Communication" Energy Center

Overview

The "communication" energy center is located at the throat and known as the "throat" chakra. This center is associated with the ability to express and communicate clear thoughts and ideas. It is also related to truth, maturity, independence and the ability to trust others. Spiritually, this center might be considered connected to "Divine Guidance." For the physical body this center can be associated with the neck, throat and jaw, vocal chords and respiratory system.

Toning

The tone for the "throat" center is the music note "G" combined with the vowel sound "eye" as in "my".

Focusing on the throat while viewing or imagining the color "blue" can enhance the toning experience for this energy center. Crystals and gemstones that could be included in the toning of this center might include lapis lazuli, blue sapphire, blue topaz, blue tourmaline and turquoise. Peppermint, spearmint, eucalyptus, sage and basil can be supportive of this chakra. The sounds of music, the outdoors, silence or a motivational speaker may aid in balance. Affirmations might include, "I always express myself truthfully and clearly," "I am able to listen when others speak," and "I am able to advocate and express my opinions easily."

Recipe

Food choices that may fortify this energy center include liquids such as water, fruit juices and herbal teas. Tart or tangy fruits such as lemons, limes and grapefruits as well as tree fruits like plums, apricots, apples, pears and peaches can be helpful here.

Seasonings include salt and lemon grass. And sea vegetables can be supportive of the thyroid.

Drinks such as water with fruit including lemon and lime have recently become very popular and it's comforting to know that they also have health benefits. Other fruits and some vegetables like cucumbers can also be added to water or herbal tea for a refreshing drink. The old fashioned remedy of rinsing the mouth and gargling with water and salt can be soothing to the "throat" center. The following recipe is also delicious.

Throat Soothing Broth

This recipe is easy to prepare either on the stove or in a crockpot. The broth can be kept warm in the crockpot, adding additional water as needed, for several days as part of a "cleanse" or light menu during recovery from an illness. It can be stored in the refrigerator and heated as needed for several days or frozen for several months. Warm broth is soothing to the throat and the vegetables provide an abundance of minerals. Please add in or leave out ingredients to your taste.

Choose a large saucepan, small stockpot or crockpot. Organic would be the best choice for this healing recipe since many of the minerals are found in the skins. Rinse all vegetables thoroughly.

Ingredients:

- Potatoes – *the whole potato or just the skins can be used; if using whole potatoes, cut into large pieces without peeling*
- Onion – *coarsely chopped, skin can be left on*
- Celery – *coarsely chopped, stalks and leaves can be used*
- Garlic - *coarsely chopped to expose the inside of the cloves*
- Parsley – *coarsely chopped, stems can be included*
- Mushrooms – *use a handful; fresh or dried; shitake, maitake, oyster, etc.*
- Kombu – *½ - 1 "stick"*

- Basil – *or other herb of choice; sometimes it is better not to include herbs if using during an illness as the taste of even your favorite herbs can seem unpleasant*
- Dark leafy greens - *coarsely chopped, stems can be included*
- Beets - *tops can be included*
- Carrots - *the whole carrot or just the skins can be used; if using whole carrots, cut into large pieces*
- Water – *cover vegetables by at least 2 inches or use up to four times the volume of vegetables*

Directions:

- Place desired vegetables in a pot of choice - *fill halfway or less*
- Add water – *see above*
- Bring to boil – *if using crockpot cook on "high"*
- Reduce heat - *for crockpot reduce to "low" for several hours or longer*
- Simmer at least 1 hour – *longer is better;*
- Strain before serving or storing – *vegetables can be discarded or composted*
- Enjoy!

intuition

"ay"

Chapter 8
"Intuition" Energy Center

Overview

The energy center that is known as the "third-eye" is located in the middle of the forehead between the eyebrows and associated with intuition and clairvoyance. This center helps us with inner guidance and attaining self-realization and is connected to imagination and awareness. Pituitary and pineal glands, nervous system, brain and skull are physical associations for this center. And not surprisingly, the eyes and vision are connected to this chakra that involves perception and insight.

Toning

The tone for the "third-eye" center is the music note "A" combined with the vowel sound "ay" as in "may" or "say".

Focus for this center would be the middle of the forehead just above eye level. Imagining or viewing the color "indigo" which is a darker version of "blue" can enhance the toning experience for this energy center. Crystals and gemstones to enhance this toning experience might include opal, blue sapphire, amethyst and tourmaline. Supporting herbs and spices include lavender, poppy seed, juniper and lemongrass. A walk under the night sky and gazing at the stars may be beneficial. Think, "I am aware in every moment, I trust my intuition!"

Recipe

Purple foods, such as blueberries, grapes, blackberries, prunes and raisins are food choices that may fortify this energy center. Versions of potatoes, cabbage and kale that are purple join eggplant as fortifiers of this third-eye chakra. Seasonings might include lavender and poppy seed, cardamom, nutmeg, turmeric and coriander. Savoring a small piece of dark chocolate or a glass of red wine very slowly might be appropriate for those who are not addicted to sugar.

Serve the recipe below with purple carrot sticks to support the chakra or enjoy with your favorite raw vegetables, pita chips or crackers.

Roasted Eggplant Dip

This recipe is a variation of a classic found in several countries and called by different names. Besides being used as a dip this eggplant mixture can be used as a salad dressing or topping for steamed vegetables. And occasionally, people have been known to eat it with a spoon.

Choose a shallow roasting pan and lightly grease with olive oil. A high speed blender or food processor would be helpful for mixing but a determined person with a masher or fork can also achieve delicious results.

Ingredients:

- 2 medium eggplants - *rinsed and dried*
- ½ cup tahini
- Lemon – *juice ½ reserving 2nd half if needed*
- ½ teaspoon sea salt
- 1 head garlic – *trim top and remove loose papery layers*
- 1 clove garlic, crushed – optional – *to be used by garlic lovers*
- 2 tablespoons olive oil – *to add to recipe*
- ½ teaspoon olive oil – *to drizzle over head of garlic*
- 1 tablespoons olive oil – *to grease roasting pan and coat eggplant*
- Fresh chopped parsley or sesame seeds for garnish

Directions:

- Heat oven to 400 degrees - *in warm weather, this recipe can be made on the grill wrapping the eggplant and garlic in aluminum foil*
- Lightly grease a shallow roasting pan
- Poke 8-10 holes in the eggplant and coat with oil allowing the oil to seep into holes
- Drizzle oil onto top of garlic and wrap with foil
- Place eggplant and garlic on baking sheet
- Check eggplant and garlic at 30 minutes and then at 10 minute intervals; both should be done in 40-60 minutes
- The eggplant is done when a skewer passes through easily and the garlic is done when soft
- Allow to cool
- Place eggplant in blender, food processor or bowl - *eggplant can be cut in large chunks leaving the skin on, especially if using a high speed blender, otherwise remove most or all of the skin and discard*
- Squeeze garlic to add to eggplant
- Add tahini, sea salt, juice of ½ lemon and crushed raw garlic if desired
- Blend until smooth
- Taste, adjust lemon adding 1 tablespoon at a time and salt if necessary
- Plate, garnish and serve
- Enjoy!

spiritual

"ee"

Chapter 9
"Spiritual" Energy Center

Overview

The seventh and final major energy center is known as the "crown" center and is located at the top of the head. Physically, it's associated with the nervous system, the brain and brain stem, spinal cord, pineal gland, and nerves. This center is connected to understanding, knowledge, wisdom and logic. And it is also the center that involves spirituality, enlightenment, and the exploration of the "meaning of life."

Toning

The tone for the "crown" center is the music note "B" combined with the vowel sound "ee" as in see.

Violet is the color to envision while toning for this "spiritual" energy center. Amethyst, quartz, and diamond can provide supporting vibrations. Supporting herbs and fragrances include lavender, sage, frankincense, myrrh, and juniper. Mountain peaks are considered to be a place of connection to this energy center, but any exposure to nature and clean air, water and sunlight could be supportive. Affirmations might include, "I connect easily with spirit" and "I am pure light and love!"

Recipe

Food choices to support the "spiritual" center could include pure, natural, organic foods that are minimally processed. Regularly eating to support the other energy centers will benefit this center as well. Fasting or detoxing might be considered to boost this center. Drinking plenty of water, juicing, sipping broth or teas and eating light meals may help this chakra to rest and regenerate.

Eat consciously. Chew slowly and thoroughly and sip rather than gulping liquids. Think about how the food you're eating is supporting your spirit. Consider replacing a meal with meditation or prayer. Breathe.

Breathing 1:

This technique, known as the "4-7-8 breath" was demonstrated by Dr. Andrew Weil at an Institute for Integrative Nutrition conference (Fall 2014) and is also available for viewing at: <u>www.drweil.com</u>

Start by practicing the technique twice a day, every day. It will soon become a tool that will be useful and available in a variety of situations. Use it when feeling stressed or anxious, before reacting to something negative that someone has said or when someone cuts you off while driving. This technique may help you to fall asleep or sidestep food cravings. Make it your newest "good habit."

Directions:

- Sit, stand or lie in a comfortable, supported posture
- Place the tip of the tongue lightly at the top of the mouth just behind the teeth and let it remain there throughout the breathing exercise
- Exhale
- Breathe in through the nose for a count of "4"
- Maintain the breath for a count of "7"
- Purse the lips as if drinking through a straw or blowing a dandelion and exhale through the mouth for a count of "8"
- Although the counts should not be rushed, the exact length of the counts is not as important as keeping them the same length relative to each other
- Complete the sequence above four times
- Enjoy!

Breathing 2:

This technique was shown to me by Nicole Cutler L.Ac., at her office in Middletown, New York. It is easiest to learn while lying face-up, but once learned it can also be done when sitting or standing. The breaths can provide increased oxygen to the body as well as being calming and centering. Only two breaths at a time are sufficient being mindful that slight dizziness is a possibility.

Directions:

- Lie face-up in a comfortable but supported position
- Place one hand weightlessly on the lower abdomen
- Exhale
- Inhale deeply with the intention of raising the hand with the breath
- Hold the breath for a few seconds
- Exhale completely
- Repeat
- Enjoy!

Chapter 10
Total Toning

Overview

Below is a chart that can be used to make toning simple:

ENERGY CENTER	COLOR	TONE	VOWEL
1 root	red	C	"uh" (cup)
2 sacral	orange	D	"ooh" (you)
3 solar plexus	yellow	E	"oh" (go)
4 heart	green	F	"ah" (ma)
5 throat	blue	G	"eye" (my)
6 third eye	indigo	A	"ay" (say)
7 crown	violet	B	"ee" (see)

Toning

Although toning can be done at any time of day, it may be beneficial to include it at the same time every day, perhaps as part of an established routine. Some people complete their practice by spending a few minutes toning the heart center and finally the root center to provide a feeling of being grounded. Others end with silent meditation and enjoy the light feeling toning may provide.

Toning may also provide a vehicle for people who have tried meditation and have felt frustrated and unsuccessful. The use of the voice, as well as multiple options for focus could provide supports to calm the mind and achieve a sense of balance.

Whether you are experiencing health challenges, interested in maintaining your current level of wellness, or just like to try new things, toning may provide you with the opportunity to use your voice to enhance your health and balance yourself.

Recipe

This recipe can contribute to all the energy centers at once. It also can provide an opportunity to get together with others, sharing food and positive energy, and perhaps toning as well.

Fruit Salad

Fresh, local, seasonal, organic fruits are the perfect ingredients for a delicious fruit salad but not always an option. Do the best you can. Include your favorites. Adding some frozen fruits can be affordable and provide a variety that would otherwise not be possible. Soaking dried fruits and then adding them to the salad can contribute a sweet quality and a variety to the texture. Citrus will help to keep the colors bright and keep the salad fresh for a few days. Decorate with a sprinkle of your favorite nuts or seeds, sprig of an herb such as mint, shredded coconut, or whipped topping of choice.

Choose a large bowl to make the salad easier to toss or if a clear bowl is available take advantage and layer the colorful fruits for a beautiful presentation.

Ingredients:

- Strawberries, raspberries, red apples, pomegranates, cherries, cranberries, watermelon
- Oranges, persimmons, tangerines, peaches, mangoes, papaya, apricots, cantaloupe, nectarines
- Yellow apples, yellow pears, pineapple, yellow figs, yellow kiwi, bananas, grapefruit
- Kiwi, green apples, green pears, green grapes, honeydew melon
- Blueberries, elderberries
- Blackberries, black currants, figs
- Purple grapes, plums

Directions:

- Choose 1-2 fruits of each color from the lists above – *include a variety of sweet and tart*
- Wash, peel or pit as needed and cut into bite sized pieces
- Place your rainbow of fruits in a bowl
- Chill and serve with chosen garnish
- Enjoy!

Conclusion

If you read and remember the Introduction to this book, I mentioned a trip with a friend. We stood next to each other during the toning session. Although the experience was very powerful and important to me, my friend was not impressed. Another example of bio-individuality.

And yet, that toning experience has contributed to my life even though it was a one-time event rather than a regular practice. Because of toning, I developed a different perspective and a new understanding of spirituality. It has enabled me to be more open to looking at many things from a different viewpoint.

When presented with the opportunity to write this book, the decision to move forward and the choice of topic were more intuitive than reasoned. The topic came to me in a dream and the decision was made. And although I have found many answers through writing, I have many more questions.

I joined a chorus when I was unable to find a group for toning and I'm wondering if toning would enhance the group energy and alignment of vowel sounds more than the traditional warm-up exercises. Would toning support team building in more traditional settings such as business, family and the classroom? Would using one's voice by toning contribute to someone being able to use their voice to advocate for themselves or others? Is your favorite song more than just a great beat that you can dance to but also a combination of tones and vibrations that literally make you "feel good"?

I think toning has something positive for everyone. Toning can support your other wellness practices, for body, mind and spirit. Give it a try. Toning may resonate with you. And you may find some answers and some questions of your own.

Sing a happy song every day.
Enjoy!

About the Author

Justine Bauer

Justine Bauer is an Institute of Integrative Nutrition Health Coach and a graduate chef of the Natural Gourmet Institute. Justine has been interested in health and nutrition for some time as a result of personal health challenges and a love of food. The belief that life and wellness are ever evolving and personal has led to an exciting and eclectic journey through many food-style and lifestyle experiments. Justine has worked in the field of children's mental health for the past sixteen years and was fortunate that facilitating trainings and presentations for parents and professionals could be included as part of the job. She recently joined a wonderful group of women participating in a Sweet Adelines International barbershop chorus "Song of the Valley." These experiences and the excitement of a new adventure have created the opportunity for Justine to write her first book, "Toning Your Life: Use Your Voice to Enhance Your Health."

http://justine-bauer.healthcoach.integrativenutrition.com/

References

"Chakra Anatomy - Discover Your Energetic Self." *Chakra Anatomy*. Web. 21 Mar. 2015.

"The Chakra Diet – Balance Your Heart Chakra and Lose Weight Too! | Metaphysics." *Before It's News*. Web. 21 Mar. 2015.

"Chakra Healing." *Charms Of Light - Healing*. Web. 21 Mar. 2015.

"Chakra Note Chart." *Sacred Waves*. Web. 21 Mar. 2015.

"Chakra System." *Natural Health Techniques*. Web. 21 Mar. 2015.

"Chakra Therapy - Balancing With Colors and Sound." *Chakra-Colors.com*. Web. 7 Dec. 2014.

"Chakra Tones." *Chakra Balancing*. Web. 7 Dec. 2014.

"Chakra Tones: Use the Power of Vocal Toning to Open and Balance the Chakras." *The Energy Healing Site*. Web. 7 Dec. 2014.

"Chakra Toning." *Sound Intentions*. Web. 7 Dec. 2014.

"Chakra Vocal Toning." *DIY Stress Relief*. Web. 7 Dec. 2014.

"Chakras, Elements, Colors and the Solfeggio Frequencies." *Soma Energetics*. Web. 7 Dec. 2014.

"Chakras." *Healing Village*. Web. 21 Mar. 2015.

"Crystals for the Root Chakra." *One -Vibration.com*. Web. 21 Mar. 2015.

Desy, Phylameana Lila. "Foods That Fuel Your Chakras." *About.com*. Web. 21 Mar. 2015.

Desy, Phylameana Lila. "Root Chakra." *About.com*. Web. 21 Mar. 2015.

Erickson, Lisa . "Food Energetics." Web. 21 Mar. 2015.

"Essential Oils for the First or Root Chakra (Muladhara)." *StarchaserHealing Artscom*. Web. 21 Mar. 2015.

"Feeding Your Chakras; Food List." *The Dao Bums*. Web. 21 Mar. 2015.

"Food for Chakra Healing." *Dahn Yoga*. Web. 21 Mar. 2015.

Henkin, Marlene. "Chakra Sound Chart." *Henkin Energy Therapy: Marlene Henkin, Integrative Therapy Healer. Reiki, Reflexology, Acupressure.* Web. 7 Dec. 2014.

Perry, Wayne. *Sound Medicine*. Fourth Printing 2012 ed. Musikarma, 2007.

"Sacral Chakra." *Crystal Meanings*. Web. 21 Mar. 2015.

"A Simple Homey, Coconut-y Red Lentil Dal." *Food52*. 02 Jan. 2014. Web. 21 Mar. 2015.

"Spiritual Affirmations for Chakras." *Chakra-Lover.com*. Web. 21 Mar. 2015.

Thompson, Jennifer. "Crystals and the Seven Chakras." *PureCalma.com*. Web. 21 Mar. 2015.

"Toning the Chakras." *Gaiam Life*. Web. 7 Dec. 2014.

Trehan, Sohini. "7 Awesome Affirmations to Balance Your Chakras." *MindBodyGreen*. 26 July 2012. Web. 21 Mar. 2015.

"Understanding Chakra Frequencies." *Chakra Healing*. Web. 7 Dec. 2014.

"Working With Your Chakras." *Soulful Healing*. 14 Oct. 2011. Web. 21 Mar. 2015.

"Your Root Chakra – Survival, Trust, Safety, and Family Loyalty - Cheri Valentine, LLC | Shamanic Healer & EFT Specialist." *Cheri Valentine LLC Shamanic Healer EFT Specialist*. 01 Mar. 2014. Web. 21 Mar. 2015.